INTERMITTENT FASTING FOR WOMEN OVER 60

ALFIE BROWN

DISCLAIMER

The information provided in this book is intended to be used for general informational purposes only. It is not a substitute for professional medical advice, diagnosis, or treatment. Always seek the advice of your physician or other qualified healthcare providers before starting any new diet or exercise regimen.

Intermittent fasting is not suitable for everyone, and it is important to consult with a healthcare professional before incorporating it into your lifestyle, especially if you have any pre-existing medical conditions or take any medications. This book is not intended to replace personalized medical advice, and the author and publisher are not liable for any injuries or health complications that may occur from following the information provided.

The author and publisher of this book make no warranties or guarantees regarding the accuracy, completeness, or usefulness of the information provided. The reader assumes full responsibility.

Thank you for choosing to read this book, and we hope that it provides valuable information and guidance on your health journey.

Table of Contents

Chapter 1: The Basics of Intermittent Fasting for Aging Women

Introduction:

Intermittent fasting, or IF, has become a popular health trend in recent years, with many people turning to this eating pattern to improve their overall health and wellbeing. It has gained even more attention in the aging community, with women over 60 seeking ways to stay healthy and vibrant as they age. In this chapter, we will discuss the basics of intermittent fasting, specifically for aging women, and how it can benefit their health.

1.1 What is intermittent fasting?

Intermittent fasting is not a diet but rather an eating pattern that cycles between periods of eating and fasting. Unlike traditional diets, IF does not focus on what you eat but rather on when you eat. It does not restrict any foods or food groups, but instead focuses on when you consume them.

There are several variations of intermittent fasting, but the most common approach is to have an eating window and a fasting window. This can range from a daily cycle of 16 hours of fasting and 8 hours of eating to longer periods of fasting, such as 24 hours once or twice a week. During the fasting window, no calories are consumed, but non-caloric beverages like water, tea, and coffee are allowed.

1.2 Benefits of Intermittent Fasting for Women Over 60

Research has shown that intermittent fasting can have numerous benefits for aging women, including:

- Improved insulin sensitivity: Insulin is a hormone that regulates blood sugar levels and can become less efficient as we age, leading to conditions like type 2 diabetes. Intermittent fasting has been shown to improve insulin sensitivity and reduce the risk of metabolic diseases.

- Increased longevity: Studies have found that intermittent fasting can increase the lifespan and healthspan of animals, and more research is being conducted on its effects on humans.

- Weight loss: A lack of physical activity and a slower metabolism can make it more challenging for women over 60 to lose weight. Intermittent fasting can help with weight loss by reducing the number of calories consumed and boosting metabolism.

- Improved cognitive function: As we age, cognitive decline and neurodegenerative diseases become more common. Intermittent fasting has been shown to improve brain function and protect against age-related cognitive decline.

- Lower inflammation levels: Chronic inflammation is linked to various health issues, and intermittent fasting has been shown to reduce inflammation levels in the body.

- Increased cellular repair: During fasting, the body goes into a cellular repair mode, getting rid of old or damaged cells and producing new ones. This process can improve overall health and may have anti-aging effects.

1.3 Who Can Benefit from Intermittent Fasting?

Intermittent fasting can be beneficial for women over 60 who want to improve their overall health and wellbeing. It can also be helpful for those who struggle with weight loss, have insulin resistance or type 2 diabetes, or are looking to combat age-related cognitive decline.

However, as with any lifestyle change, it is essential to consult with a doctor before starting intermittent fasting, particularly if you have any underlying health conditions or take medications that need to be taken with food.

1.4 Understanding the Different Types of Intermittent Fasting

There are several different types of intermittent fasting, each with its unique approach. The most common ones include:

- The 16/8 method - This involves fasting for 16 hours and having an 8-hour eating window every day.
- The 5:2 diet - This approach involves eating normally for 5 days a week and limiting calorie intake to 500-600 calories on the remaining two days.
- Alternate-day fasting - This method involves fasting every other day, with some variations allowing for 500-600 calories on fasting days.
- The Warrior Diet - This involves a 20-hour fast followed by a 4-hour eating window every day.
- The OMAD (one meal a day) diet - This method involves fasting for 23 hours and having one meal within a 1-hour eating window each day.

1.5 How to Get Started with Intermittent Fasting

Before starting intermittent fasting, it is essential to determine which approach works best for you and your lifestyle. It is also crucial to consult with a doctor, particularly if you have any underlying health conditions.

To get started, it's best to ease into intermittent fasting gradually. Start by extending the time between your meals, then gradually reduce your eating window until you reach your desired fasting period. It is also essential to listen to your body and adjust the fasting periods if you feel unwell.

In the next chapter, we will delve deeper into the benefits of intermittent fasting for aging women, including its effects on specific health conditions and its impact on overall quality of life. Now that you have a basic understanding of intermittent fasting, you can begin to explore this eating pattern and its potential benefits for your health and wellbeing.

Chapter 2: Preparing for Intermittent Fasting

Intermittent fasting has gained popularity in recent years as a way to improve overall health and aid in weight loss. However, before jumping into this eating pattern, it is important to prepare your body and mind for the changes that come with fasting. In this chapter, we will discuss the steps that should be taken to properly prepare for intermittent fasting.

2.1 Consulting with a Healthcare Professional

Before starting any new diet or eating plan, it is crucial to consult with a healthcare professional. This is especially important for individuals with pre-existing health conditions or those taking medication, as intermittent fasting may affect their health differently. A healthcare professional can evaluate your overall health and provide personalized recommendations and guidance for starting intermittent fasting.

Additionally, individuals with a history of disordered eating or restrictive eating habits should also consult with a healthcare professional before beginning intermittent fasting. Fasting can sometimes trigger unhealthy behaviors for those with a history of disordered eating and it is important to approach it with caution and proper guidance.

2.2 Setting Realistic Goals

Setting realistic goals before beginning intermittent fasting can help you stay motivated and on track. This could include goals such as weight loss, improved energy levels, or better digestion. By setting achievable goals, you will have a clear focus and purpose for implementing this eating pattern.

It is important to note that intermittent fasting is not a quick fix for weight loss or a magic solution for health. It should be seen as a long-term lifestyle change that requires patience and dedication. Setting unrealistic expectations can lead to disappointment and a higher likelihood of giving up on the plan.

2.3 Choosing the Right Intermittent Fasting Plan

There are several different types of intermittent fasting plans, each with their own unique benefits and challenges. It is important to choose the plan that best fits your lifestyle and aligns with your goals. Some popular options include the 16:8 method, the 5:2 diet, and alternate day fasting.

The 16:8 method involves fasting for 16 hours and having an 8-hour eating window each day. The 5:2 diet involves eating normally for five days and restricting calorie intake to 500-600 calories on two non-consecutive days. Alternate day fasting involves fasting every other day and eating normally on non-fasting days.

Consider your schedule, energy levels, and potential food restrictions when choosing which intermittent fasting plan to follow. It may also be helpful to experiment with different plans to find the one that works best for you.

2.4 Creating a Meal Plan

Once you have chosen your intermittent fasting plan, it is important to create a meal plan. This will help you stay on track and make sure you are consuming healthy, nutritious meals during your eating window. It is crucial to include a variety of foods from all food groups to ensure you are getting all the necessary nutrients.

During fasting periods, it is important to stay hydrated by drinking plenty of water, herbal teas, and other non-caloric beverages. Planning and preparing meals in advance can also help reduce the temptation to break a fast with unhealthy foods.

2.5 Getting Your Body Ready for Fasting

Before starting your intermittent fasting plan, it is helpful to get your body ready for the upcoming changes. This could include gradually reducing your calorie intake or practicing short periods of fasting to prepare your body for longer fasting periods.

It is also important to prioritize healthy habits such as regular exercise and getting enough sleep. These habits can help support your body during the fasting period and improve overall health.

In conclusion, proper preparation is essential before starting any new eating pattern, including intermittent fasting. Consulting with a healthcare professional, setting realistic goals, choosing the right plan, creating a meal plan, and getting your body ready for fasting are all crucial steps for a successful intermittent fasting journey. By taking these steps, you can ensure a safe and sustainable approach to intermittent fasting for improved health and well-being.

Chapter 3: How to Start Intermittent Fasting

Intermittent fasting is a popular method of eating that involves alternating periods of fasting and eating within a specific time frame. It has gained a lot of attention in recent years due to its potential health benefits, including weight loss, improved blood sugar control, and increased energy.

If you are new to intermittent fasting, getting started can seem intimidating. But with the right approach and guidance, it can be a simple and rewarding experience. In this chapter, we will discuss the key steps to successfully starting intermittent fasting and staying on track towards your health goals.

3.1 Choosing a Start Date

The first step to starting intermittent fasting is choosing a start date. It's important to set a specific date and commit to it, rather than just saying "I'll start eventually." This will help you mentally prepare and make the necessary adjustments to your schedule.

When choosing a start date, consider your schedule and lifestyle. If you have a busy week ahead, it may not be the best time to start fasting as it can be challenging to manage hunger and cravings when you are occupied and stressed. Instead, pick a time when you can devote more attention to your eating habits and fasting routine.

Additionally, it's a good idea to start on a weekend or a day off from work. This will allow you to get used to fasting without the pressure of being surrounded by co-workers or feeling the need to explain your new eating habits.

3.2 Fasting Schedule and Duration

There are various methods of intermittent fasting, such as the 16/8 method, the 5:2 method, and the alternate-day fasting method. As a beginner, it's best to start with a more manageable approach, such as the 16/8 method. With this method, you fast for 16 hours and have an 8-hour eating window.

Some people may prefer to start with a shorter fasting period, such as 12 hours, and slowly increase their fasting duration as they get more comfortable. Experiment with different schedules to find what works best for you.

Also, consider when you'll be breaking your fast. It's usually recommended to have your first meal in the late morning or early afternoon to align with your body's circadian rhythm. This will make it easier to maintain your fasting schedule in the long run.

3.3 Tips for Managing Hunger and Cravings

During the fasting period, you may experience hunger pangs and cravings for food. This is normal and expected, especially when you are first starting. However, there are a few tips that can help you manage these sensations and stay on track with your fast:

- Stay hydrated: Drinking water, black coffee, and tea can help suppress hunger and keep you feeling full.
- Stay busy: Keeping yourself occupied with work, hobbies, or exercise can help keep your mind off food.
- Chew gum or snack on low-calorie foods: Chewing gum or snacking on small amounts of low-calorie foods like fruits and vegetables can also help curb hunger and cravings.

It's also essential to listen to your body. If you are feeling weak, dizzy, or lightheaded, it may be a sign that you need to break your fast and eat something.

3.4 Dealing with Social Pressures

Intermittent fasting is a personal choice, and you may encounter some social pressures from friends, family, or co-workers who may not understand or agree with your decision. They may question why you're not eating with them or try to convince you to break your fast.

It's essential to stay committed to your goals and not let outside influences sway you. Educate those around you about the potential benefits of intermittent fasting and explain your reasons for doing it. You can also suggest alternative social activities that don't revolve around food, such as going for a walk or watching a movie.

Remember, your health and well-being should always come first, and it's okay to politely decline offers of food or explain your eating habits to others.

3.5 Staying Motivated to Continue Fasting

As with any new habit, staying motivated can be a challenge. To stay committed to intermittent fasting, it's helpful to have a clear understanding of your goals and why you chose to start this journey. Whether it's for weight loss, improved health, or more energy, remind yourself of these reasons whenever you feel like giving up.

Additionally, track your progress to see how far you've come and celebrate any milestones or achievements along the way. Surround yourself with a support system of friends or online groups who are also practicing intermittent fasting. They can provide encouragement, accountability, and helpful tips to stay on track.

Conclusion:

Starting intermittent fasting may seem daunting at first, but with the right approach and mindset, it can be a sustainable and beneficial way of eating. Choose a start date, determine your fasting schedule and duration, learn how to manage hunger and cravings, deal with social pressures, and stay motivated. With consistency and patience, you can reap the potential health benefits of intermittent fasting and achieve your wellness goals.

Chapter 4: Maximizing Health Benefits while Fasting

Fasting has been practiced for centuries as a way to improve physical, mental, and spiritual health. It is a powerful tool for promoting weight loss, improving insulin sensitivity, and reducing inflammation in the body. However, fasting can also have its risks if not done properly, especially for women over 60. In this chapter, we will discuss how to maximize the health benefits of fasting while ensuring that it is safe for older women.

4.1 Hydration and Nutrition

One of the most important factors to consider when fasting is hydration. It is essential to drink enough water throughout the day to prevent dehydration, which can lead to dizziness, fatigue, and other health problems. For women over 60, it is recommended to drink at least eight glasses of water per day, even when fasting. Avoiding sugary drinks or artificially sweetened beverages is also crucial for maintaining good health while fasting.

In addition to water, it is essential to ensure that you are getting proper nutrition while fasting. This is especially important for women over 60, as they may already have nutritional deficiencies due to age and other factors. During fasting, it is recommended to consume nutrient-dense foods such as leafy greens, lean protein, and healthy fats to support your body's needs. Incorporating bone broth, green juice, and herbal tea can also provide essential vitamins and minerals.

4.2 Supplements for Women Over 60

Supplements can be beneficial for women over 60 who are fasting, as they can help fill in any nutritional gaps. However, it is essential to consult with a healthcare professional before taking any supplements, as they may interact with medications or have adverse effects. Some supplements that can be beneficial during fasting include omega-3 fatty acids, vitamin D, and probiotics.

Omega-3 fatty acids are crucial for brain health and reducing inflammation in the body. Vitamin D is essential for maintaining strong bones, and probiotics can help support a healthy gut microbiome.

4.3 Exercise Recommendations

Exercise is an essential component of maintaining good health, especially during fasting. However, it is essential to find a balance between exercising enough to promote health benefits, but not overdoing it and causing fatigue or injury. For women over 60, low-impact exercises such as walking, yoga, or swimming may be more appropriate than high-intensity workouts.

It is also essential to listen to your body when exercising while fasting. If you feel lightheaded, dizzy, or have any discomfort, it is essential to stop and rest. It is better to take it easy and gradually increase exercise intensity as your body adjusts to fasting.

4.4 Monitoring Your Health while Fasting

It is crucial to listen to your body and monitor your health while fasting, especially if you are a woman over 60. Pay attention to any signs of dehydration, such as thirst, dry mouth, or dark urine, and drink more water if necessary. It is also vital to monitor your blood sugar levels regularly, especially if you have diabetes or prediabetes.

If you experience any adverse effects while fasting, such as extreme fatigue, dizziness, or weakness, it is important to break your fast and consult with your doctor.

4.5 Dealing with Medications and Intermittent Fasting

For women over 60, it is common to take various medications for managing health conditions. When incorporating intermittent fasting into your lifestyle, it is essential to consult with your doctor or healthcare provider first, as fasting can affect the absorption and effectiveness of certain medications.

It is crucial to take medications as prescribed and not skip doses while fasting. If you experience any adverse side effects, consult with your doctor immediately. They may be able to adjust your medication schedule or recommend other alternatives to ensure your safety and well-being while fasting.

In conclusion, fasting can be a valuable tool for improving health and well-being for women over 60. By staying hydrated, maintaining proper nutrition, and monitoring your health, you can safely reap the benefits of fasting and promote longevity and overall wellness. As always, it is essential to listen to your body and consult with your doctor before making any significant changes to your diet or exercise routine.

Chapter 5: Dealing with Potential Challenges

Intermittent fasting is a powerful tool for improving overall health and reaching weight loss goals. However, embarking on an intermittent fasting journey may bring about potential challenges that can hinder progress and discourage individuals from sticking to their fasting schedule. In this chapter, we will discuss some common obstacles that people may face when practicing intermittent fasting, as well as provide strategies for overcoming them.

5.1 Overcoming Common Obstacles

One of the most common obstacles that people face when practicing intermittent fasting is hunger. During the fasting period, the body may send signals of hunger, which can be difficult to ignore. To overcome this challenge, it is essential to stay hydrated, as thirst may be misinterpreted as hunger. Drinking plenty of water and staying hydrated can help curb hunger and keep you feeling full.

Another obstacle that people may face is cravings. When practicing intermittent fasting, individuals may have a limited eating window, which may lead to cravings for certain foods. To overcome this, it is important to keep healthy snacks within reach during the eating window. This can include fruits, vegetables, nuts, and seeds. Preparing healthy meals and snacks ahead of time can also help in avoiding unhealthy food cravings.

5.2 Dealing with Stress and Emotional Eating

Stress and emotions can play a significant role in our eating habits. Many people turn to food for comfort when dealing with stress or negative emotions, which can sabotage the intermittent fasting journey. It is vital to develop strategies for dealing with stress and emotions without resorting to food. This can include practicing relaxation techniques like yoga or meditation, journaling, or talking to a trusted friend or therapist. Finding alternative ways to cope with stress and emotions can help avoid overeating during fasting periods.

5.3 Avoiding Overeating during Eating Windows

One of the potential challenges of intermittent fasting is overeating during the eating window. It is important to remember that intermittent fasting is not an excuse to eat whatever and however much you want during the eating window. Overeating can lead to consuming more calories than necessary, which can hinder weight loss progress. To avoid overeating, it is important to practice mindful eating. This means paying attention to your body's fullness cues and stopping when you feel satisfied, rather than stuffed. It may also be helpful to plan and prepare your meals in advance, ensuring that they are well-balanced and nutrient-dense.

5.4 Strategies for Breaking a Fast

Breaking a fast properly is essential to avoid discomfort and digestive issues. When breaking a fast, it is important to start with easily digestible foods such as fruits, vegetables, and soups. Avoiding heavy and processed foods can help ease the digestive system back into eating. It is also essential to hydrate and drink plenty of water throughout the eating window.

5.5 Addressing Negative Reactions from Others

Lastly, one of the potential challenges of intermittent fasting is receiving negative reactions from others. Intermittent fasting may be a new concept to some people, and they may have misconceptions or doubts about its effectiveness or safety. It is important to be confident in your decision to practice intermittent fasting and explain its benefits and how it works to those who may question it. Surrounding yourself with a supportive community of like-minded individuals can also help in navigating any negative reactions from others.

In conclusion, intermittent fasting can bring about potential challenges, but with the right strategies and mindset, these obstacles can be overcome. It is essential to stay hydrated, plan and prepare meals, find alternative ways to cope with stress and emotions, practice mindful eating, and properly break a fast. By addressing these potential challenges and having the right tools and resources, individuals can successfully stick to their intermittent fasting journey and reach their health and weight loss goals.

Chapter 6: Long-term Success with Intermittent Fasting

In the previous chapters, we have discussed the numerous health benefits of intermittent fasting, including weight loss, improved metabolic health, and increased longevity. However, to truly reap the long-term benefits of intermittent fasting, it is important to find sustainable and personalized strategies that work for you as an individual.

In this chapter, we will focus on long-term success with intermittent fasting, specifically for aging women. As we age, our bodies and nutritional needs change, and it is crucial to adapt our fasting practices accordingly. We will also explore the mental and emotional aspects related to maintaining a healthy lifestyle and celebrating successes along the way.

6.1 Maintenance Strategies for Aging Women

Intermittent fasting is not a quick-fix solution; it is a long-term lifestyle change that requires consistency and dedication. As we age, our metabolism tends to slow down, making weight loss and weight maintenance more challenging. This is why it is crucial for aging women to find maintenance strategies that work for their bodies and lifestyles.

The first step in maintaining your intermittent fasting practice is to understand your body's unique needs and limitations. As women age, we experience hormonal changes and a decrease in muscle mass, both of which can affect our metabolism. It is important to consult with a healthcare professional to ensure your fasting practices are safe and sustainable.

Additionally, as we age, our nutritional needs also change. It is important to focus on incorporating nutrient-dense foods into your diet, such as lean proteins, healthy fats, and complex carbohydrates. These foods will provide your body with the necessary nutrients for optimal health and help you maintain your weight loss.

6.2 Adapting Fasting as You Age

It is crucial to be open to adapting your fasting practice as you age. Our bodies are dynamic, and what works for us in our 20s may not be as effective in our 50s. As we mentioned before, consulting with a healthcare professional can help you determine the best approach for your specific needs.

One adaptation you may need to make is adjusting your fasting window. As we age, our bodies may not be able to handle long periods without food, and it may be necessary to shorten your fasting window or incorporate occasional breaks from fasting. You can also experiment with different types of intermittent fasting, such as alternate-day fasting or time-restricted eating, to find what works best for your body.

6.3 Creating a sustainable lifestyle

Intermittent fasting is not just about weight loss; it is about creating a sustainable lifestyle. This means finding a balance between your fasting and eating windows and incorporating healthy habits into your daily routine. It is important to listen to your body's signals and not restrict yourself too much, as this can lead to yo-yo dieting and an unhealthy relationship with food.

One way to create a sustainable lifestyle is to meal prep and plan your meals ahead of time. This will help you stay on track with your fasting and make healthier food choices. Also, find ways to make intermittent fasting enjoyable, such as trying new recipes, incorporating different types of workouts, and including social activities during your eating window.

6.4 Tracking Progress and Adjusting as Needed

Tracking your progress is crucial for long-term success with intermittent fasting. This includes keeping track of your weight, body measurements, and how you feel overall. It is essential to note any changes or improvements you notice, such as increased energy levels, improved sleep, or improved digestion.

It is also important to have a flexible mindset and be open to adjusting your fasting practice as needed. If you notice a plateau in weight loss, or if your body is not responding well to a certain fasting schedule, it may be time to reassess and make changes accordingly. Remember, intermittent fasting is not a one-size-fits-all approach, and it is important to listen to your body and make adjustments as needed.

6.5 Celebrating and Maintaining Weight Loss

Weight loss is a significant achievement, and it is important to celebrate your successes along the way. However, it is equally important to focus on maintaining your weight loss. This can be done by continuing with your fasting practice, incorporating regular physical activity, and making healthy food choices.

It is also important to be aware of potential triggers and be mindful of your emotions and stress levels. Sometimes, emotional or stress eating can lead to weight regain, so finding healthy coping mechanisms and support systems is crucial for maintaining your weight loss.

6.6 *The Mental and Emotional Aspect of Long-term Success with Intermittent Fasting*

Intermittent fasting is not just about the physical changes, but also the mental and emotional changes that come with it. As women, we are often bombarded with unrealistic beauty standards, which can take a toll on our mental and emotional well-being.

Intermittent fasting provides an opportunity to not only improve our physical health but also our relationship with food. It teaches us to listen to our bodies and trust their signals, rather than adhering to strict diets. It also allows for a healthier balance between indulging in treats and maintaining a nutritious diet.

It is important to practice self-love and body positivity while on your intermittent fasting journey. Celebrate your progress, and don't be too hard on yourself when things don't go as planned. Always remember that health and happiness should be the ultimate goals.

In conclusion, long-term success with intermittent fasting for aging women requires a combination of understanding your body's changing needs, adapting your fasting practice accordingly, creating a sustainable lifestyle, tracking progress, and prioritizing mental and emotional well-being. By following these strategies and making adjustments as needed, you can experience the full benefits of intermittent fasting and maintain a healthy lifestyle for the long term. Remember to always consult with a healthcare professional before making any significant changes to your diet and fasting practices.

Conclusion

In this book, we have discussed the unique challenges and experiences that women over 60 face and how to navigate through this stage of life with health and vitality. It is essential to remember that age is just a number, and with the right mindset and lifestyle, we can continue to thrive and enjoy all that life has to offer.

Throughout the book, we have focused on the importance of self-care, including maintaining a healthy diet, staying physically active, taking care of our mental health, and finding ways to fulfill our passions and purpose. These pillars of self-care are crucial for women over 60, as they can help improve overall well-being and quality of life.

We have also touched upon the physical and hormonal changes that occur during this stage of life, and how to manage them through proper nutrition, exercise, and sometimes medication or supplements. It is essential to understand and embrace these changes and work with our bodies to continue living our best lives.

Moreover, we have emphasized the importance of building a strong support system, whether it be family, friends, or community groups. Having a support system is crucial for our mental and emotional well-being, especially during this stage of life when we may face challenges such as retirement, empty nest syndrome, or loss of loved ones.

As we age, it is also important to stay connected and engaged in the world around us, whether it be through social activities, volunteering, or pursuing hobbies and interests. Continuously learning and growing can help us stay mentally sharp and fulfill us on a deeper level.

In conclusion, this book has been a guide for women over 60 to embrace their age gracefully and live their best lives. It is a reminder that age should not limit us, but instead, it is an opportunity to continue growing, learning, and thriving. By prioritizing self-care, building a support system, and staying connected and engaged, we can navigate through this stage of life with vitality and joy.

Additional Resources for Women Over 60:

1. Ageless Women, Timeless Wisdom: Lessons from Remarkable Women by Lois P. Frankel, Carol A. Osborne, and Kim A. Pacini (2004)

2. The Wisdom of Menopause: Creating Physical and Emotional Health and Healing During the Change (Revised Edition), by Christiane Northrup, MD (2006)

3. The Confidence Code: The Science and Art of Self-Assurance – What Women Should Know by Katty Kay and Claire Shipman (2014)

4. The Power of Meaning: Crafting a Life That Matters by Emily Esfahani Smith (2017)

5. The Art of Growing Old: A Guide to Aging with Grace by Marie De Hennezel (2012)

Appendix: Meal Plan Examples

Meal Plan 1:
- Breakfast: Avocado toast with whole grain bread, topped with scrambled eggs and spinach
- Snack: Greek yogurt with berries and almonds
- Lunch: Quinoa and black bean salad with mixed greens and a lemon vinaigrette dressing
- Snack: Apple slices with almond butter
- Dinner: Baked salmon with roasted vegetables and whole grain couscous
- Dessert: Dark chocolate-covered strawberries

Meal Plan 2:
- Breakfast: Overnight oats with almond milk, chia seeds, and mixed berries
- Snack: Hummus and veggie sticks
- Lunch: Turkey and avocado wrap with whole wheat tortilla, served with a side of fruit
- Snack: Whole grain crackers with cheese
- Dinner: Grilled chicken with roasted sweet potatoes and steamed broccoli
- Dessert: Baked apples with cinnamon and Greek yogurt

Appendix: Exercise Recommendations for Women Over 60

It is recommended for women over 60 to engage in at least 150 minutes of moderate-intensity aerobic activity (such as brisk walking, swimming, or cycling) every week. This can easily be broken down into 30 minutes of exercise, 5 days a week.

In addition to aerobic exercise, it is also important to incorporate strength training into your routine, which can help maintain muscle mass and bone density. Strength training can include using weights, resistance bands, or bodyweight exercises.

Here are some exercise recommendations for women over 60 to consider:

1. Walking or jogging: This low-impact aerobic exercise is great for cardiovascular health and can be easily modified based on your fitness level.

2. Yoga or Pilates: These exercises focus on balance, strength, and flexibility and can help improve mobility and reduce the risk of falls.

3. Water aerobics: This low-impact exercise is gentle on the joints and can provide a full-body workout.

4. Cycling: Whether it's on a stationary bike or outdoors, cycling is a great way to get a cardio workout and build leg strength.

5. Dancing: Not only is dancing fun, but it also provides a great cardiovascular workout and can improve balance and coordination.

6. Strength training: Incorporating strength training into your routine is important for maintaining muscle mass and bone health. Consider using weights, resistance bands, or bodyweight exercises.

Remember to always listen to your body and take breaks when needed. It is also important to consult with a healthcare professional before starting any new exercise routine, especially if you have any medical conditions. Lastly, make sure to stay hydrated and properly fuel your body with nutritious foods for optimal energy during exercise.